Wall Pilates Workouts for Women Over 60

Age is Just a Number, Feel Amazing with Wall Pilates

Helen Talbott

Disclaimer:

The information contained in this book is for educational purposes only and is not intended as a substitute for professional medical advice, diagnosis, or treatment. Always consult with a qualified healthcare professional before starting any new exercise program, especially if you have any pre-existing medical conditions.

The author and publisher disclaim any liability for any adverse effects resulting from the use of the information contained in this book.

The author and publisher of this book have made every effort to ensure the accuracy and completeness of the information provided. However, the information contained herein is for educational purposes only and is not intended as a substitute for professional medical advice, diagnosis, or treatment.

Always consult with a qualified healthcare professional before starting any new exercise program, especially if you have any pre-existing medical conditions.

The author and publisher disclaim any liability for any adverse effects arising from the use of the information contained in this book.

Limitations of Information:

The information provided in this book is based on the author's knowledge and experience, as well as current research on Wall Pilates and exercise for older adults. However, individual results may vary, and what works for one person may not work for another.

It is important to listen to your body, modify exercises as needed, and stop if you experience any pain or discomfort.

Medical Disclaimer

This book is not intended to diagnose or treat any medical condition. If you have any concerns about your health, please consult with a doctor or other qualified healthcare professional.

Warranty Disclaimer

The author and publisher make no warranties, expressed or implied, with respect to the accuracy, completeness, or effectiveness of the information contained in this book.

Copyright and Intellectual Property Disclaimer

All materials contained in this book are protected by copyright and other intellectual property laws. You may not reproduce, distribute, or modify any part of this book without the written permission of the author.

About the Author

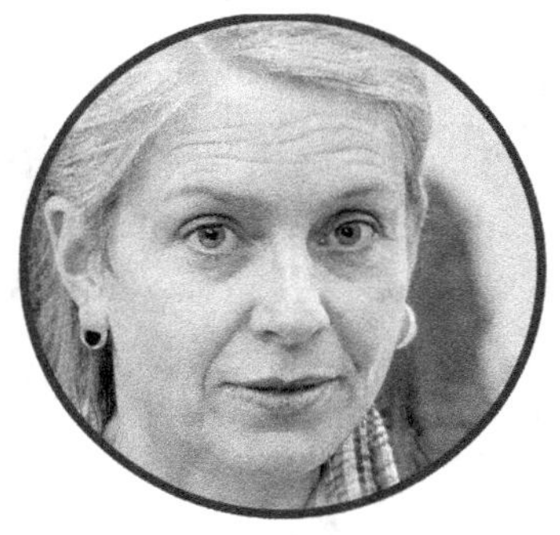

Helen Talbott is a passionate advocate for health and well-being, Driven by a belief that age is just a number, she embarked on a personal journey to discover ways to maintain strength, flexibility, and vitality even in later years. This led her to the transformative world of Wall Pilates, a gentle yet effective practice that became the foundation of her own fitness routine.

Inspired by its benefits, Helen felt compelled to share her newfound passion with others. With a background in fitness and healthcare, she delved deeper into the practice, acquiring certifications and refining her knowledge. Witnessing firsthand the positive impact Wall Pilates had on women in her community fueled her desire to create a comprehensive guide specifically tailored for their needs.

"Age is Just a Number, Feel Amazing with Wall Pilates Workouts for Women Over 60" is the culmination of Helen's personal journey and dedication to empower others. Her writing reflects her warm, encouraging, and relatable approach, making complex exercises accessible and motivating. She believes that every woman, regardless of age or fitness level, can unlock their inner strength and experience the joy of movement through Wall Pilates.

Table of contents

Introduction

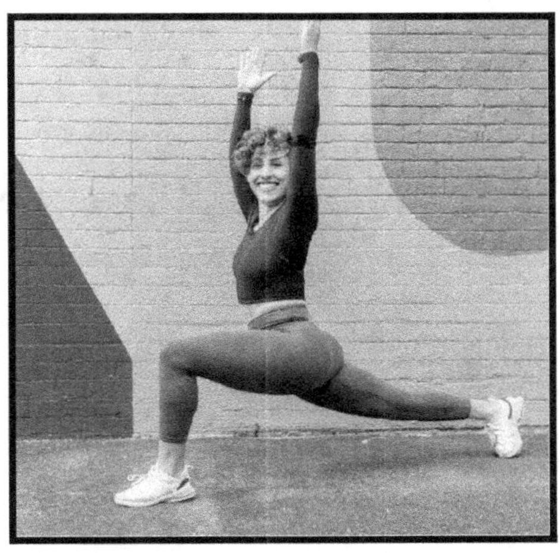

Welcome to Your Fitness Rejuvenation: Why Wall Pilates After 60?

Sixty. It's not just a number, it's a milestone often shrouded in misconceptions and societal expectations. But what if this milestone wasn't an ending, but rather a **vibrant new beginning**?

Welcome to **Redefine Sixty: Age is Just a Number, Feel Amazing with Wall Pilates**, your guide to unlocking a **fitness renaissance** in your post-60s journey. Forget the stereotypes; this isn't about chasing lost youth, but about **embracing a powerful, confident version of yourself**.

Why Wall Pilates?

Forget intimidating gyms and high-impact routines. Wall Pilates offers a **gentle yet effective** fitness practice specifically designed for the changing needs of your body after 60. Imagine:

- **Strength & stability:** Sculpt and tone muscles, **improving balance and reducing fall risk**.
- **Pain management:** Ease joint discomfort and stiffness, promoting pain-free movement.
- **Flexibility & mobility:** Stay agile and limber, allowing you to navigate daily life with ease.

- **Bone health:** Build stronger bones to combat osteoporosis and maintain healthy posture.
- **Stress relief & improved sleep:** Unwind and de-stress, boosting your energy and overall well-being.

More than just physical benefits:

Wall Pilates isn't just about exercise; it's about **empowering yourself**. This book will guide you through:

- **Understanding your body:** Learn about the unique changes associated with aging and how to tailor workouts accordingly.
- **Mastering the fundamentals:** Discover the core principles of Pilates, ensuring proper form and maximizing results.
- **Crafting personalized workouts:** Choose routines that match your fitness level and address your specific concerns.
- **Staying motivated and inspired:** Find tips and strategies to build a sustainable practice and celebrate your progress.

Embrace the possibilities:

Redefining sixty isn't just about feeling physically amazing; it's about **rediscovering your spirit of adventure and possibility**. This book is your invitation to join a community of women on a shared journey of **strength, empowerment, and joyful living**. So, take a deep breath, step onto your mat, and get ready to redefine what it means to be sixty and beyond.

Are you ready to embark on this transformative journey? Let's begin!

Debunking Myths and Reframing Our Perspective on Aging

Society often paints aging with a negative brush, filled with limitations and decline. But what if those limitations are largely myths? Let's break down some common misconceptions and shift our perspective towards a more empowering and positive view of aging:

Myth 1: You lose muscle mass and strength inevitably.

Reality: While some decline is natural, regular exercise, especially strength training like Pilates, can **combat muscle loss and even build new muscle**, increasing strength and power well into your golden years.

Myth 2: Exercise becomes too difficult or dangerous after 60.

Reality: This myth overlooks the beauty of **adaptability and personalized exercise**. Wall Pilates offers modifications and gentle movements that can be effective and safe for various fitness levels and limitations.

Myth 3: Aging means physical and mental decline.

Reality: The brain maintains amazing neuroplasticity throughout life, meaning it can continue to learn and grow. Staying physically active stimulates brain health, boosting memory, cognitive function, and mood.

Myth 4: Your life slows down and becomes less exciting after 60.

Reality: This is your chance to explore new passions, travel, connect with loved ones, and pursue adventures without the constraints of earlier commitments. Embrace this time of freedom and self-discovery!

Reframing Our Perspective:

Shifting our mindset about aging is crucial for embracing its potential. Here's how to reframe your perspective:

- **Focus on resilience and growth:** See aging as a time to develop new skills, overcome challenges, and build inner strength.
- **Celebrate experience and wisdom:** Your years hold valuable knowledge and lessons, making you a unique and insightful individual.
- **Embrace change as an opportunity:** Adapt to physical changes with grace and discover the joy of trying new things.
- **Prioritize your well-being:** Self-care, healthy habits, and meaningful connections are key to thriving in any decade.

By debunking myths and reframing our perspective, we can unlock a vibrant and fulfilling second chapter of life. Remember, age is just a number, and the power to redefine your possibilities lies within you. Let's move away from limitations and embrace the exciting journey of aging with strength, wisdom, and boundless joy!

What to Expect From This Book: Your Roadmap to Feeling Amazing

Welcome to your personal guide to reclaiming your **strength, health, and vitality** after 60! This book is your roadmap to a **transformed you**, using the gentle yet powerful practice of Wall Pilates. Forget the limitations and negativity often associated with aging – here, you'll discover a path to **feeling amazing, both physically and mentally**.

What's inside:

- **Foundations for Success:** We'll lay the groundwork with an understanding of your changing body, essential Pilates principles, and tips for creating a safe and comfortable practice space.
- **Personalized Workouts:** No two bodies are alike, and neither are your goals! We'll offer a variety of **tailored workouts** addressing strength, flexibility, common concerns like joint pain and bone health, and even stress management.

- **Clear Guidance and Support:** Each exercise comes with **detailed instructions, modifications, and visual aids**, ensuring you perform them safely and effectively.
- **Motivational Inspiration:** Get ready for tips on staying motivated, building a sustainable practice, and celebrating your progress along the way.
- **Beyond the Mat:** We'll explore how to integrate healthy habits into your lifestyle, connect with a supportive community, and discover resources for further learning and exploration.

What you'll achieve:

- **Improved strength and balance:** Move with confidence and reduce your risk of falls.
- **Enhanced flexibility and mobility:** Stay agile and navigate daily life with ease.
- **Reduced pain and improved joint health:** Feel better and move freely.

- **Stronger bones and improved posture:** Combat osteoporosis and maintain a healthy frame.
- **Reduced stress and improved sleep:** Boost your energy and overall well-being.
- **Increased confidence and empowerment:** Reclaim your sense of self and embrace your inner strength.

Remember:

This journey is **not about chasing lost youth**. It's about **discovering a new, empowered version of yourself**, one that thrives on movement, vitality, and self-care. This book is your supportive guide, offering the knowledge, tools, and motivation you need to **redefine what it means to be 60 and beyond**.

So, are you ready to embark on this transformative journey? Let's begin!

I hope this helps! Feel free to ask me any questions you may have.

Chapter 1

Understanding Your Body After 60: Changes, Considerations, and Individualization

Sixty and beyond is a vibrant and exciting chapter, yet your body undergoes several changes compared to earlier decades. Understanding these changes is crucial for creating a safe and effective Wall Pilates practice designed specifically for your needs.

Key Changes to Be Aware Of:

- **Muscle Mass & Strength:** Muscle mass naturally declines with age, impacting strength and stamina. However, regular exercise, like Wall Pilates, can slow down this decline and even build new muscle.
- **Bone Density:** Bone density starts to decrease after menopause, increasing the risk of osteoporosis. Weight-bearing

exercises like Wall Pilates can help maintain bone health and strength.

- **Flexibility & Balance:** Joints may become less flexible, and balance may decline due to various factors. Gentle stretches and balance exercises in Wall Pilates can improve both.
- **Metabolic Rate:** Your metabolism may slow down, making it easier to gain weight and harder to lose it. Staying active with Wall Pilates helps manage weight and boost metabolism.
- **Sensory & Cognitive Changes:** Vision, hearing, and reaction times may subtly change. Modifications and clear instructions in Wall Pilates ensure safety and effectiveness.

Individualization is Key:

Remember, **every body is unique**. These changes may vary in their intensity and timeline. Here's how to personalize your practice:

- **Listen to your body:** Pay attention to any pain or discomfort and adjust exercises accordingly. Don't push yourself beyond your limits.
- **Consult your doctor:** Before starting any new exercise program, discuss it with your doctor, especially if you have any health conditions.
- **Start slowly and gradually progress:** Begin with low-impact exercises and gradually increase intensity and duration as you build strength and confidence.
- **Modify exercises:** Don't hesitate to modify exercises to suit your limitations. Many variations and adaptations are possible within Wall Pilates.
- **Focus on quality over quantity:** Proper form and controlled movements are more important than speed or repetitions.

Embrace Your Unique Journey:

Aging is a natural process, and your body's changing needs are simply part of the adventure. By understanding these changes and prioritizing individualized exercises, you can leverage Wall Pilates to not only **maintain your health and well-being but also thrive in your 60s and beyond**.

Chapter 2

Essential Wall Pilates Principles: Alignment, Breath, Flow, and Control

Welcome to the cornerstone of your Wall Pilates practice! In this chapter, we'll explore the four fundamental principles that guide every movement, ensuring **safety, effectiveness, and ultimate success**. These principles are your compass, navigating you towards a practice that strengthens, energizes, and empowers you.

1. Alignment: Your Body's Strong Foundation:

Imagine your body as a magnificent building. Proper alignment ensures its stability and strength. In Wall Pilates, alignment focuses on:

- **Neutral spine:** Maintain a natural S-curve, avoiding slouching or arching your back.

- **Engaged core:** Activate your deep abdominal muscles for support and stability.
- **Balanced posture:** Distribute your weight evenly across your feet and avoid leaning on one side.
- **Long neck and head:** Align your head with your spine, avoiding tension in the neck and jaw.

Remember, perfect alignment isn't about rigidity; it's about finding a comfortable, balanced position that supports optimal movement.

2. Breath: Fueling Your Movements:

Breath isn't just about staying alive; it's the lifeblood of your Pilates practice. In Wall Pilates, we use:

- **Controlled, coordinated breathing:** Inhale through your nose and exhale through your mouth, synchronizing breath with movement.

- **Deep diaphragmatic breathing:** Engage your diaphragm for deeper breaths, maximizing oxygen intake and improving core engagement.
- **Rhythm and flow:** Match your breath to the flow of each exercise, creating a sense of connection and control.

Remember, mindful breathing helps deliver oxygen to your muscles, fuels your movements, and reduces stress.

3. Flow: Moving with Grace and Intention:

Imagine a dancer gliding seamlessly across the stage. That's the essence of flow in Wall Pilates. We strive for:

- **Smooth transitions:** Connect each movement with controlled transitions, avoiding jerky motions.
- **Continuous movement:** Maintain momentum throughout the exercises, creating a sense of continuous flow.

- **Mind-body connection:** Focus on your muscles and how they move, ensuring each movement is intentional and controlled.

Remember, graceful flow prevents injuries, maximizes muscle engagement, and makes your practice enjoyable and meditative.

4. Control: Power with Precision:

Control isn't about pushing yourself to the limit; it's about precision and focus. In Wall Pilates, we emphasize:

- **Slow and controlled movements:** Avoid rushing through exercises; every movement should be deliberate and controlled.
- **Focus on quality over quantity:** Prioritize perfect form over repetition; fewer perfect repetitions are more effective than numerous rushed ones.
- **Listen to your body:** If you feel strain or pain, modify the exercise or take a break.

Remember, controlled movements ensure safety, maximize muscle activation, and build strength and stability effectively.

Embracing the Whole:

These four principles are interconnected and weave together to create the magic of Wall Pilates. By consciously focusing on **alignment, breath, flow, and control**, you move beyond mere repetitions and transform your practice into a mindful, transformative experience.

Remember, consistency and practice are key. As you integrate these principles, you'll not only achieve your fitness goals but also cultivate a deeper mind-body connection, leaving you feeling stronger, more balanced, and ready to embrace life with renewed vitality.

Chapter 3

Gearing Up: Equipment, Clothing, and Setting Up Your Practice Space

Welcome to your personalized Pilates studio! While Wall Pilates requires minimal equipment, preparing your space and choosing the right attire can significantly enhance your experience. Let's explore the essentials to set you up for success:

Essential Equipment:

- **A sturdy wall:** Your reliable workout partner! Choose a smooth, clear space on a wall you can comfortably use for various exercises.
- **A yoga mat:** Your comfortable landing pad. Opt for a non-slip mat with ample cushioning for joint protection.
- **Optional extras:** Depending on your goals and preferences, you may consider:

- **Light hand weights:** Add resistance for strength training. Choose weights you can lift with good form.
- **Resistance bands:** Offer versatile options for adding resistance to various exercises.
- **Pilates ball:** Great for core strengthening and balance challenges.
- **Ankle weights:** Target lower body strengthening for specific goals.

Remember: Safety first! Choose equipment appropriate for your fitness level and consult your doctor if you have any health concerns.

Clothing for Comfort and Movement:

- **Breathable, comfortable clothing:** Opt for clothes that allow for full range of motion, like leggings and loose-fitting tops.

- **Supportive footwear:** Wear well-fitting socks or comfortable shoes with good grip, like yoga socks or barefoot shoes.
- **Optional extras:**
  - **Headband or hair tie:** Keep your hair out of your face for distraction-free movement.
  - **Water bottle:** Stay hydrated throughout your practice.

Creating Your Sanctuary:

- **Clear a spacious area:** Ensure you have enough room to move freely and safely without bumping into furniture or walls.
- **Good lighting and ventilation:** Choose a well-lit and well-ventilated space for a pleasant and comfortable environment.
- **Minimize distractions:** Turn off phones or televisions to stay focused on your practice. Consider calming music if it enhances your experience.
- **Personalize your space:** Add elements that inspire you, like motivational quotes or pictures of loved ones.

Remember: Your practice space is your personal haven. Customize it to reflect your individual needs and preferences, making it a place you look forward to stepping into for your daily dose of invigorating Wall Pilates!

Chapter 4

Safety First: Modifications and Tips for Avoiding Injuries

Your journey towards a stronger, healthier you with Wall Pilates starts with safety. This chapter equips you with the knowledge and tools to prevent injuries and ensure a safe and enjoyable practice.

Understanding Your Limits:

Remember, **listening to your body is crucial**. It's okay to modify exercises or take breaks if you feel pain, discomfort, or fatigue. Pushing through pain can lead to injuries, hindering your progress.

Common Sense Safety Tips:

- **Warm-up and cool down:** Prepare your body with gentle stretches and light cardio before each workout, and wind down with relaxing stretches afterward.

- **Start slow and progress gradually:** Don't try to do too much too soon. Begin with beginner-friendly exercises and gradually increase intensity and duration as you build strength and confidence.
- **Maintain proper form:** Pay attention to alignment, breath, and control in every movement. Don't compromise form for speed or repetitions.
- **Listen to your doctor:** If you have any health conditions, consult your doctor before starting a new exercise program.
- **Use proper equipment:** Ensure you choose equipment that fits your body and fitness level.

Modifications for Every Body:

Wall Pilates offers immense flexibility for individual needs. Here are some common modifications you can incorporate:

- **Reduce range of motion:** If an exercise feels too challenging, shorten the movement or decrease the angle of your body.

- **Use props for support:** Use a chair, wall, or yoga block for balance and stability.
- **Reduce weight or resistance:** If using weights or resistance bands, choose lighter options or modify the exercises to reduce tension.
- **Skip exercises that cause pain:** Don't force yourself through pain. There are always alternative exercises that target similar muscle groups.

Additional Tips:

- **Focus on quality over quantity:** It's better to perform fewer exercises with perfect form than many with compromised technique.
- **Stay hydrated:** Drink plenty of water before, during, and after your workout.
- **Rest and recover:** Allow your body time to rest and recover between workouts.

- **Seek professional guidance:** If you're unsure about an exercise or modification, consult a qualified Pilates instructor.

Remember: Safety is paramount. By incorporating these tips and modifications, you create a personalized practice that works for your unique body and abilities, allowing you to reap the benefits of Wall Pilates while minimizing the risk of injury.

Chapter 5

Energize Your Mornings: Gentle Wake-Up Flow

Start your day on a vibrant note with this **gentle Wake-Up Flow**. Designed to energize your body and mind, this sequence of Wall Pilates exercises will leave you feeling refreshed, focused, and ready to embrace the day.

Benefits:

- **Improved circulation and mobility**
- **Increased energy levels and reduced fatigue**
- **Enhanced mood and reduced stress**
- **Gentle stretching and strengthening for major muscle groups**
- **Improved balance and coordination**

Preparation:

Before you begin, find a quiet space with a sturdy wall and your yoga mat. Wear comfortable clothing that allows for full range of motion. Choose calming music if desired.

The Flow:

1. Wall Cat-Cows (5 repetitions each direction):

- Stand facing the wall with your hands shoulder-width apart and fingertips lightly touching the wall.

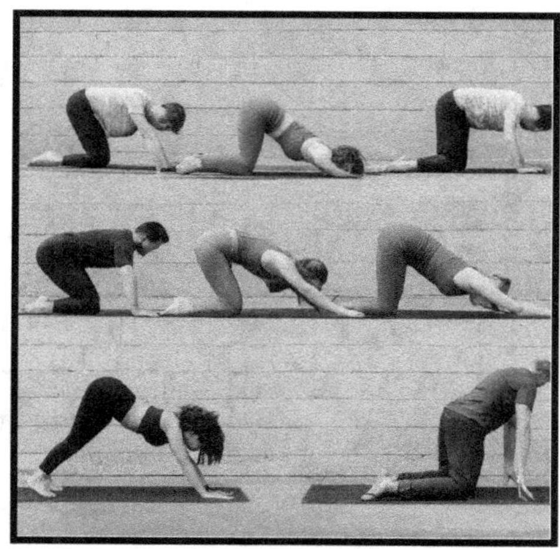

- Inhale as you arch your back, dropping your belly button towards the floor and gazing upwards.

- Exhale as you round your spine, drawing your belly button towards your spine and tucking your chin towards your chest.
- Flow smoothly between these movements, focusing on your breath and spinal articulation.

2. Wall Sun Salutations (3 repetitions):

- Stand facing the wall with your feet hip-width apart.

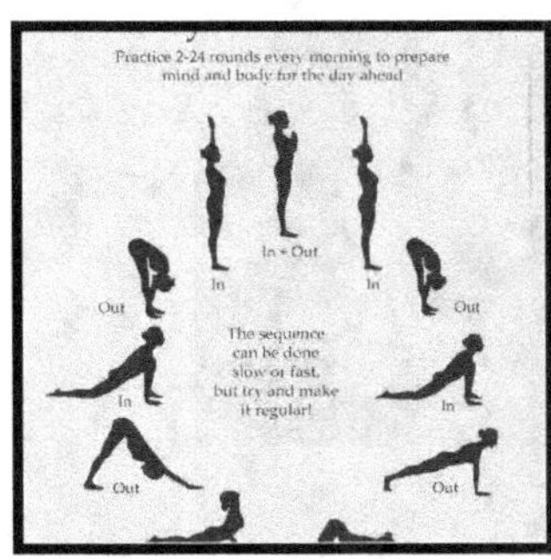

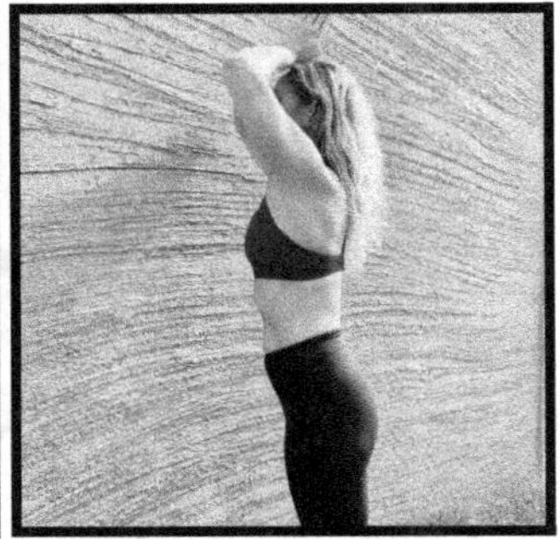

- Inhale as you raise your arms overhead, fingertips touching the wall.
- Exhale as you step back from the wall, placing your hands shoulder-width apart on the wall, and bending forward, lengthening your spine.

- Inhale as you lift your torso and hips parallel to the floor, gazing forwards.
- Exhale as you step back towards the wall, returning to the standing position with arms raised overhead.

3. Wall Leg Lifts (10 repetitions each leg):

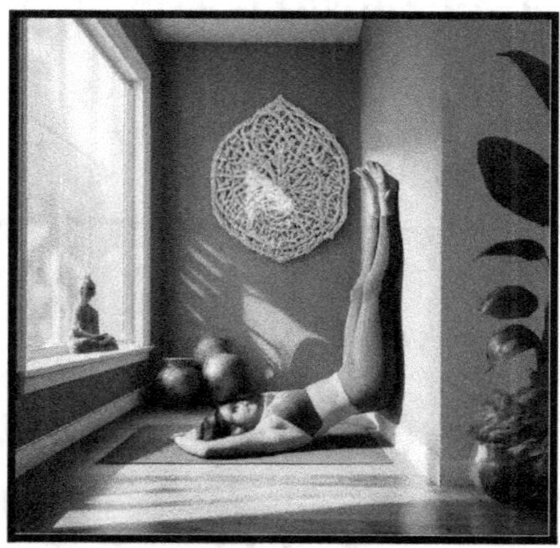

- Stand sideways facing the wall with your hand closest to the wall on the wall for support.
- Extend your other leg straight back, parallel to the floor.
- Inhale as you lift your straight leg up towards the ceiling.

- Exhale as you slowly lower your leg back down.
- Repeat with the other leg.

4. Wall Push-Ups (Modification options offered below):

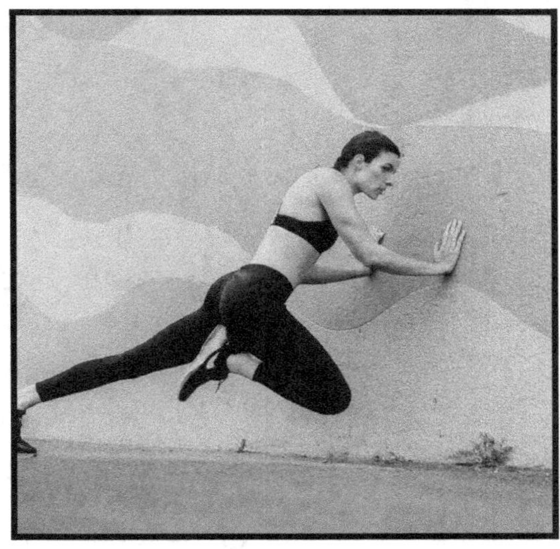

- Stand facing the wall with your feet hip-width apart and hands placed slightly wider than shoulder-width apart on the wall.

- Bend your elbows and lower your chest towards the wall, keeping your core engaged and back straight.
- Use your arms to press back up to the starting position.

Modification options:

- Perform push-ups on your knees instead of toes.
- Incline your body further away from the wall for a less challenging option.
- Use lighter weights in your hands for added resistance.

5. Wall Side Stretches (10 breaths each side):

- Stand sideways facing the wall with your arm closest to the wall extended up and hand touching the wall.
- Place your other hand on your hip.
- Lean onto the wall, stretching your side body and reaching your hand overhead if possible.

- Hold for 10 breaths, then repeat on the other side.

6. Wall Roll-Downs (5 repetitions):

- Stand facing the wall with your feet hip-width apart and hands resting on the wall at shoulder height.
- Inhale as you slowly roll down your spine, one vertebra at a time, until your hands reach your lower legs.
- Exhale as you slowly roll back up, stacking your vertebrae one at a time.

Cool Down:

- Spend a few minutes sitting or lying down with gentle stretches and deep breaths.

Remember:

- Listen to your body and modify exercises as needed.
- Focus on your breath and mindful movement.

- Celebrate your progress and enjoy the invigorating energy this flow brings to your mornings!

Additional Notes:

- You can adapt this flow to your fitness level by adjusting the number of repetitions or sets.
- Consider adding calming music or essential oils to enhance the meditative aspect of the practice.
- Encourage journaling or affirmations after your flow to set positive intentions for your day.

Chapter 6

Sculpt and Tone: Full-Body Wall Pilates Workout

Ready to elevate your fitness routine and sculpt a stronger, more toned physique? This **powerful Full-Body Wall Pilates Workout** targets major muscle groups while challenging your balance and coordination. Embrace the burn and feel the confidence boost as you build strength and definition throughout your entire body.

Benefits:

- Improved muscle tone and definition in arms, legs, core, and glutes
- Increased strength and endurance
- Enhanced balance and stability
- Boosted metabolism and calorie burning
- Enhanced body awareness and posture

Preparation:

Find a clear space with a sturdy wall and your yoga mat. Wear comfortable, form-fitting clothing that allows full range of motion. Prepare light weights (optional) and a water bottle. Choose upbeat music if desired.

The Workout:

Warm-Up (5 minutes):

- Gentle jumping jacks or jumping rope
- Arm circles (forward and backward)
- Shoulder rolls
- Dynamic stretches for legs and torso

Strength & Sculpting (3 sets of 10-12 repetitions each exercise):

1. Wall Squats:

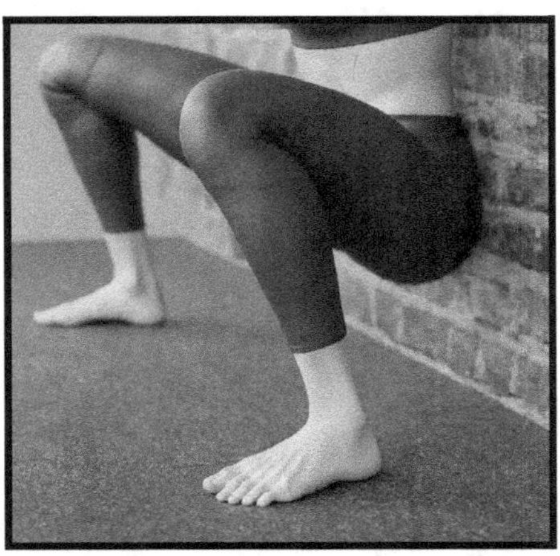

- Stand with your back against the wall, feet hip-width apart, and toes slightly outward.
- Slide down the wall as if sitting into a chair, keeping your core engaged and back straight.
- Push through your heels to return to standing.
- **Modification:** Perform squats without the wall or use a chair for support.

2. Wall Push-Ups (with variations):

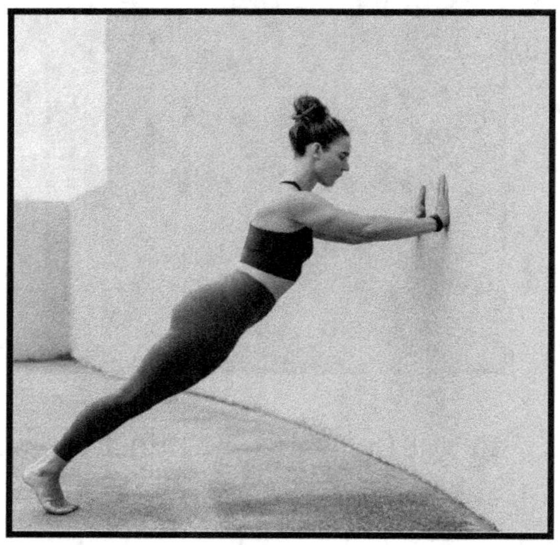

- Place your hands slightly wider than shoulder-width apart on the wall, feet hip-width apart.
- Lower your chest towards the wall, keeping your core engaged and back straight.
- Push back up to starting position.

- **Modification:** Perform push-ups on your knees or incline your body further away from the wall for a less challenging option.

3. Wall Lunges:

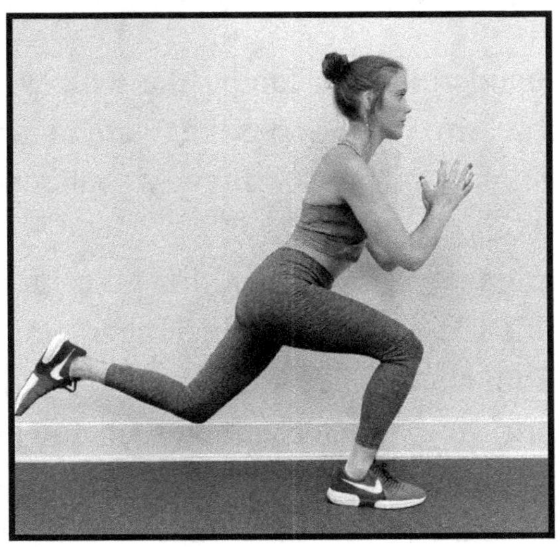

- Stand with your back against the wall, one leg forward and other leg extended back with toes on the floor.
- Lower your body, bending both knees, until your front knee forms a 90-degree

angle and your back knee hovers near the floor.

- Push through your front heel to return to standing.
- Repeat with the other leg.

4. Wall Side Plank with Leg Lifts:

- Stand sideways facing the wall with your forearm resting on the wall at shoulder height, elbow directly under your shoulder.
- Engage your core and lift your hips into a side plank position, forming a straight line from head to heels.
- Lift your top leg straight up towards the ceiling and lower back down.
- Repeat with the other leg.

5. Wall Tricep Dips:

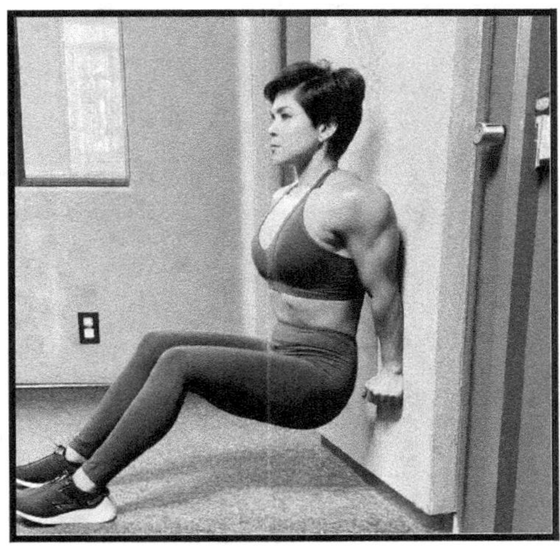

- Sit on the floor with your back against the wall, hands shoulder-width apart behind you, fingertips facing forward.
- Walk your feet out until your legs are straight and form a 90-degree angle with your torso.
- Lower your body by bending your elbows, keeping your back close to the wall.
- Push back up to starting position.

Cool Down (5 minutes):

- Gentle stretches for major muscle groups
- Deep breathing exercises

Remember:

- Modify exercises as needed and listen to your body.
- Maintain proper form and controlled movements.
- Push yourself, but don't compromise form for speed or repetitions.
- Focus on your breath and connect with your body throughout the workout.
- Celebrate your progress and enjoy the empowering feeling of sculpting a stronger, fitter you!

Additional Notes:

- Consider adding ankle weights or light dumbbells for further resistance.
- Offer alternative exercises for those with any limitations or injuries.
- Encourage recording your progress and setting achievable goals to stay motivated.

I hope this helps!

Chapter 7

Enhance Flexibility and Balance: Stretching and Stability Exercises

Maintaining flexibility and balance are crucial aspects of healthy aging and overall well-being. This chapter presents a dynamic blend of **gentle stretches and targeted stability exercises** designed to improve your range of motion, enhance coordination, and prevent falls.

Benefits:

- Increased flexibility and range of motion in major muscle groups
- Improved balance and coordination for everyday activities
- Reduced risk of falls and injuries
- Enhanced posture and body awareness
- Increased blood flow and circulation

Preparation:

Find a clear space with enough room to move freely and a yoga mat or comfortable surface. Wear loose-fitting clothing that allows for full range of motion. Choose calming music if desired.

Stretching Sequence (10-15 breaths each stretch):

1. **Hamstring Stretch:** Sit on the floor with legs extended, and reach for your toes or shins, keeping your back straight. Focus on lengthening your spine and relaxing your hamstrings.

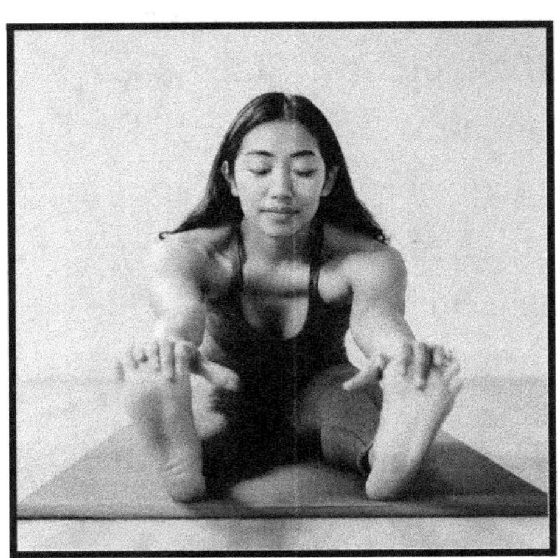

2. **Quadriceps Stretch:** Lie on your stomach, bend one leg into your chest, and hold your foot with your hand. Gently pull your heel towards your buttocks, drawing your quadriceps muscle.
3. **Chest Stretch:** Stand or sit tall, interlace your fingers behind your back and gently press your palms outwards, stretching your chest and shoulders.
4. **Neck Stretches:** Slowly tilt your head to one side, bringing your ear towards your shoulder. Hold, then repeat on the other side. Gently roll your head in a circular motion, forward and backward.
5. **Calf Stretches:** Stand facing a wall with your hands on the wall for support. Step one leg back, keeping your heel flat on the floor. Lean into the wall, feeling the stretch in your calf muscle. Repeat with the other leg.

Stability Exercises (3 sets of 10-12 repetitions each):

1. **Single-Leg Wall Stands:** Stand facing the wall with your hands lightly touching the wall for support. Lift one leg off the floor and hold for a few seconds. Maintain a tall posture and engage your core. Repeat with the other leg.

2. **Heel-Toe Walk:** Walk forward on your tiptoes for a few steps, then switch to walking on your heels. Repeat this sequence, focusing on maintaining balance and control.

3. **Side Plank with Leg Lifts:** Lie on your side with your elbow directly under your shoulder and forearm on the floor. Lift your hips into a side plank position, forming a straight line from head to heels. Extend your top leg straight up and lower back down. Repeat with the other leg.

4. **Tree Pose:** Stand tall on one leg, bringing your other foot to rest on your inner calf or ankle. Hold for a few seconds, keeping your hips square and engaging your core. Repeat with the other leg.

5. **Chair Squats:** Sit back as if sitting into an imaginary chair, keeping your back straight and heels flat on the floor. Hold for a few seconds before pushing through your heels to return to standing.

Cool Down (5 minutes):

- Gentle stretches for major muscle groups
- Deep breathing exercises

Remember:

- Breathe deeply throughout the exercises.
- Prioritize proper form over speed or repetitions.
- Modify exercises as needed to suit your limitations.
- Focus on feeling the stretches and engaging the targeted muscles.
- Celebrate your progress, even small improvements make a difference!

Chapter 8

Joint Care and Pain Management: Exercises for Back, Hips, and Knees

Living with joint pain, especially in crucial areas like your back, hips, and knees, can significantly impact your mobility and quality of life. This chapter offers **gentle yet effective exercises** specifically designed to improve joint health, manage pain, and increase your overall well-being.

Benefits:

- Reduced pain and stiffness in back, hips, and knees
- Improved joint mobility and flexibility
- Increased strength and stability around the joints
- Enhanced posture and body awareness
- Improved circulation and reduced inflammation

Preparation:

Find a clear space with enough room to move freely and a yoga mat or comfortable surface. Wear loose-fitting clothing that allows for full range of motion. Have light weights (optional) and a water bottle ready. Choose calming music if desired.

Important Note:

It's crucial to consult your doctor or a qualified healthcare professional before starting any new exercise program, especially if you have existing joint pain or medical conditions. They can advise on modifications and ensure your safety during your practice.

Gentle Exercises for Back, Hips, and Knees:

Back:

- **Cat-Cow Poses:** On all fours, arch your back as you inhale (cow) and round your back as you exhale (cat). Repeat gently, focusing on spinal mobility.

- **Seated Spinal Twists:** Sit on the floor with legs extended, twist your upper body to one side, gently looking over your shoulder. Hold for a few breaths, then repeat on the other side.
- **Bird-Dog:** On all fours, extend one arm and opposite leg simultaneously, keeping your back flat and engaged core. Hold for a few breaths, then repeat on the other side.

Hips:

- **Wall Hip Slides:** Stand sideways facing a wall with your hands on the wall for support. Slide your leg up the wall as high as comfortable, keeping your core engaged. Hold for a few breaths, then lower your leg and repeat on the other side.
- **Clamshell:** Lie on your side with knees bent and stacked. Lift your top knee slightly off the ground, keeping your hips stacked. Hold for a few breaths, then lower and repeat on the other side.

- **Glute Bridge:** Lie on your back with knees bent and feet flat on the floor. Lift your hips off the ground, squeezing your glutes. Hold for a few breaths, then lower and repeat.

Knees:

- **Straight Leg Raises:** Lie on your back with one leg extended straight up. Gently lift your leg a few inches off the ground, hold for a few breaths, then lower and repeat with the other leg.
- **Knee Circles:** Sit on a chair with feet flat on the floor. Slowly draw small circles with one knee, first in one direction then the other. Repeat with the other knee.
- **Heel Slides:** Sit on a chair with your feet flat on the floor. Slide your heel forward and back along the floor, keeping your leg straight. Repeat with the other leg.

Additional Tips:

- Modify exercises based on your pain level and abilities.
- Use props like pillows or rolled-up towels for added support.
- Listen to your body and take breaks as needed.
- Focus on quality of movement over number of repetitions.
- Combine these exercises with gentle stretches and heat therapy for additional relief.

Remember:

Managing joint pain is a journey, not a quick fix. Be patient, consistent, and celebrate small improvements. Wall Pilates can be a powerful tool in your journey towards pain-free and active living.

Chapter 9

Boost Bone Health and Prevent Falls: Osteoporosis-Focused Wall Pilates

Osteoporosis, characterized by weakened bones, poses a significant challenge for many, increasing the risk of fractures and falls. This chapter specifically addresses this concern, guiding you through **modified Wall Pilates exercises** designed to **enhance bone mineral density, improve balance, and reduce your risk of falls.**

Benefits:

- Increased bone mineral density in weight-bearing areas like hips, spine, and wrists
- Improved muscle strength and balance, reducing the risk of falls

- Enhanced coordination and agility for everyday activities
- Reduced pain and improved flexibility
- Increased confidence and independence in daily life

Preparation:

Find a clear space with a sturdy wall and your yoga mat. Wear loose-fitting, comfortable clothing that allows for full range of motion. Have light weights (optional) and a water bottle ready. Choose calming music if desired.

Important Note:

Consult your doctor before starting this program, especially if you have been diagnosed with osteoporosis or have any concerns about your bone health. They can advise on personalized modifications and ensure your safety.

Osteoporosis-Focused Wall Pilates Exercises:

Weight-Bearing Exercises:

- **Wall Squats:** Stand with your back against the wall, feet hip-width apart, and toes slightly outward. Slowly lower yourself down as if sitting into a chair, keeping your core engaged and back straight. Push through your heels to return to standing.

- **Wall Lunges:** Stand sideways facing the wall with one leg forward and other leg extended back with toes on the floor. Lower your body, bending both knees, until your front knee forms a 90-degree angle and your back knee hovers near the floor. Push through your front heel to return to standing. Repeat with the other leg.

- **Heel Raises:** Stand facing the wall with your hands on the wall for support. Rise up onto your tiptoes, hold for a few seconds, and slowly lower back down.

Balance and Coordination Exercises:

- **Single-Leg Wall Stands:** Stand facing the wall with your hands lightly touching the wall for support. Lift one leg off the floor and hold for a few seconds. Maintain a tall posture and engage your core. Repeat with the other leg.

- **Side Plank with Leg Lifts:** Lie on your side with your elbow directly under your shoulder and forearm on the floor. Lift your hips into a side plank position, forming a straight line from head to heels. Extend your top leg straight up and lower back down. Repeat with the other leg.
- **Heel-Toe Walk:** Walk forward on your tiptoes for a few steps, then switch to walking on your heels. Repeat this sequence, focusing on maintaining balance and control.

Additional Tips:

- Modify exercises to match your fitness level and limitations.
- Use light weights for added resistance, but prioritize proper form over heavy weights.
- Focus on controlled movements and deep breaths during each exercise.

- Be consistent with your practice for optimal results.
- Combine these exercises with a healthy diet rich in calcium and vitamin D for improved bone health.

Remember:

Wall Pilates is a valuable tool in supporting bone health and reducing the risk of falls. By being mindful, consistent, and consulting your doctor, you can empower yourself to live an active and independent life despite osteoporosis.

Additional Notes:

- Include visuals or illustrations demonstrating safe and effective modifications for these exercises.
- Offer resources for finding osteoporosis support groups or communities for additional guidance and motivation.
- Encourage mindfulness practices like meditation or deep breathing to manage stress and promote overall well-being.

I hope this helps!

Chapter 10

Enhance Energy and Improve Sleep: Pilates for Stress Relief and Relaxation

In today's fast-paced world, chronic stress can significantly impact our physical and mental well-being. This chapter delves into the power of **Pilates for stress relief and relaxation**, guiding you through a sequence of gentle exercises designed to:

- **Reduce stress hormones and anxiety**
- **Improve sleep quality and duration**
- **Promote relaxation and inner peace**
- **Boost energy levels and combat fatigue**
- **Enhance mood and overall well-being**

Preparation:

Find a quiet space with a sturdy wall and your yoga mat. Wear comfortable, loose-fitting clothing that allows for full range of motion. Prepare calming music (optional) and a lavender-scented candle or essential oil diffuser (optional) to create a serene atmosphere.

Gentle Exercises for Stress Relief and Relaxation:

1. Cat-Cow Poses:

- Begin on all fours with your hands shoulder-width apart and knees hip-width apart.
- As you inhale, arch your back, dropping your belly button towards the floor and gazing upwards (cow pose).
- As you exhale, round your back, drawing your belly button towards your spine and tucking your chin towards your chest (cat pose).

- Flow smoothly between these movements, focusing on your breath and spinal articulation.

2. Wall Hamstring Stretches:

- Stand facing the wall with your hands shoulder-width apart and fingertips lightly touching the wall.
- Extend one leg straight back, heel flat on the floor.
- Keeping your back straight and standing tall, gently lean into the wall, feeling the stretch in your hamstring.
- Hold for 10-15 breaths, then repeat with the other leg.

3. Seated Spinal Twists:

- Sit on the floor with your legs extended in front of you.
- Bend your knees and bring your feet flat on the floor.
- Place your hands behind you, fingertips pointing outwards.

- Gently twist your upper body to one side, looking over your shoulder.
- Hold for 5-10 breaths, then repeat on the other side.

4. Child's Pose:

- Kneel on the floor with your toes together and knees hip-width apart.
- Sit back on your heels and rest your forehead on the floor or a pillow.
- Extend your arms forward with your palms flat on the floor.
- Breathe deeply and allow your body to relax completely.
- Hold for as long as desired.

5. Supine Leg Lifts:

- Lie on your back with your knees bent and feet flat on the floor.
- Slowly extend one leg straight up towards the ceiling, keeping your core engaged and back flat on the mat.

- Hold for a few breaths, then lower your leg and repeat with the other leg.

Additional Tips:

- Modify exercises as needed based on your comfort level.
- Focus on your breath and mindful movement throughout the practice.
- Practice these exercises regularly for optimal results.
- Combine these exercises with other relaxation techniques like meditation or deep breathing for enhanced stress relief.
- Create a relaxing bedtime routine to promote better sleep.

Remember:

Pilates is a powerful tool for managing stress and promoting relaxation. By incorporating these gentle exercises into your routine, you can cultivate inner peace, improve sleep quality, and boost your overall well-being.

Chapter 11

Nutrition and Lifestyle Tips for Optimal Results

Fueling your body and mind properly is crucial to maximizing the benefits of your Wall Pilates practice and achieving optimal results. This chapter delves into essential **nutrition and lifestyle tips** that will complement your workouts and support your overall well-being.

Nourishing Your Body:

- **Balanced Diet:** Focus on whole, unprocessed foods from all food groups – fruits, vegetables, whole grains, lean protein, and healthy fats. Aim for a variety of colors on your plate for a diverse range of nutrients.
- **Hydration:** Water is essential for optimal health and performance. Aim to drink plenty of water throughout the day, especially before, during, and after your workouts.

- **Mindful Eating:** Practice mindful eating to develop a healthy relationship with food. Savor your meals, avoid distractions, and listen to your body's hunger and fullness cues.
- **Post-Workout Nutrition:** Replenish your energy stores with a balanced snack or meal containing carbohydrates and protein within 30 minutes of your workout.

Enhancing Your Lifestyle:

- **Sufficient Sleep:** Aim for 7-8 hours of quality sleep each night to allow your body to recover and rebuild muscle. Establish a relaxing bedtime routine and create a sleep-conducive environment.
- **Stress Management:** Chronic stress can hinder your progress. Practice stress-management techniques like deep breathing, meditation, or yoga to find inner peace and improve your overall well-being.
- **Movement Throughout the Day:** Don't be a couch potato! Integrate movement

into your daily routine through activities like walking, taking the stairs, or stretching.

- **Positive Mindset:** Cultivate a positive attitude and self-compassion. Celebrate your achievements, focus on progress, and believe in your ability to reach your goals.

Additional Tips:

- Consult a registered dietitian for personalized nutrition guidance tailored to your needs and goals.
- Explore healthy and delicious recipes incorporating Wall Pilates-friendly ingredients.
- Find an accountability partner or join a fitness community for support and motivation.
- Track your progress and celebrate your milestones to stay inspired.

Remember:

Making small, sustainable changes in your diet and lifestyle can significantly impact your health and well-being. By combining healthy eating habits with your Wall Pilates practice, you'll empower yourself to achieve optimal results and live a vibrant, fulfilling life.

Additional Notes:

- Consider including sample meal plans or snack ideas specifically suited for Wall Pilates practitioners.
- Offer resources for finding qualified registered dietitians or nutritionists.
- Share inspiring stories of individuals who have transformed their lives through Wall Pilates and healthy lifestyle choices.
- Emphasize the importance of listening to your body and making adjustments as needed to ensure a safe and enjoyable practice.

I hope this helps!

Chapter 12

Staying Motivated and Building a Sustainable Practice

Congratulations! You've embarked on your Wall Pilates journey, explored various exercises, and learned about its benefits for your body and mind. Now comes the key: **staying motivated and building a sustainable practice**. This chapter equips you with the tools and mindset to keep moving, embrace progress, and make Wall Pilates a cherished part of your life.

Understanding Motivation:

Motivation fluctuates. Recognize that there will be days when you feel energized and days when dragging yourself to the mat seems impossible. Understanding these ebbs and flows is crucial for navigating your journey.

Tips for Staying Motivated:

- **Set SMART goals:** Specific, Measurable, Achievable, Relevant, and Time-bound goals keep you focused and provide a sense of accomplishment.
- **Find an accountability partner:** Share your goals and progress with a friend or family member for support and encouragement.
- **Track your progress:** Use a journal, app, or progress photos to celebrate milestones and visualize your journey.
- **Focus on progress, not perfection:** Celebrate small wins and remember that even small steps contribute to long-term success.
- **Make it fun!:** Explore different Wall Pilates variations, choose upbeat music, or practice outdoors for a refreshing change.
- **Reward yourself:** Celebrate achievements with non-food rewards like a relaxing bath, a new workout outfit, or an activity you enjoy.

Building Sustainability:

- **Schedule your workouts:** Treat your practice like important appointments and block out time in your calendar.
- **Start small and gradually increase:** Begin with shorter sessions and gradually increase duration and intensity as you build stamina.
- **Find a convenient space:** Dedicate a corner in your home or find a nearby park for an easily accessible practice space.
- **Adapt to your lifestyle:** If life gets busy, opt for shorter, more frequent sessions instead of lengthy workouts you can't fit in.
- **Listen to your body:** Take rest days when needed and modify exercises to prevent injuries.
- **Join a community:** Connect with other Wall Pilates enthusiasts online or in-person for shared motivation and support.

Remember:

Building a sustainable practice is a journey, not a sprint. Be patient with yourself, celebrate progress over perfection, and find joy in the movement. Wall Pilates is a gift you give to yourself, empowering you to live a healthier, happier, and more fulfilling life.

Chapter 13

Celebrating Your Progress and Connecting with a Community: Your Journey Continues

You've come a long way! By embracing Wall Pilates, you've invested in your strength, flexibility, and well-being. Now, it's time to **acknowledge your achievements, connect with others, and continue thriving on your journey**.

Celebrating Your Progress:

- **Reflect on your journey:** Take a moment to appreciate how far you've come. Think about how you feel stronger, more flexible, or have improved your balance.
- **Acknowledge your milestones:** Did you overcome a challenging exercise? Did you increase your workout duration? Celebrate every win, big or small.

- **Reward yourself:** Treat yourself to something special, like a relaxing massage, a new workout outfit, or a healthy meal you enjoy.
- **Track your progress:** Use photos, journals, or fitness trackers to visualize your journey and stay motivated.
- **Share your success:** Tell your friends, family, or online community about your achievements. Share your story to inspire others!

Connecting with a Community:

- **Find your tribe:** Connect with other Wall Pilates enthusiasts online or in-person. Look for forums, social media groups, or local classes.
- **Share your experiences:** Offer and receive support, tips, and motivation from others on the same journey.
- **Find an accountability partner:** Team up with someone who shares your goals and can encourage you on your good and bad days.

- **Participate in challenges or events:** Look for online or local Wall Pilates challenges or events to stay motivated and connect with others.
- **Seek inspiration:** Follow experienced Wall Pilates practitioners or instructors for guidance and motivation.

Beyond the Mat:

- **Integrate movement into your daily life:** Take the stairs, park further away, or do quick stretches throughout the day.
- **Nourish your body:** Eat healthy foods that fuel your workouts and overall well-being.
- **Prioritize sleep:** Aim for 7-8 hours of quality sleep to allow your body to recover and rebuild.
- **Manage stress:** Practice relaxation techniques like meditation, deep breathing, or spending time in nature.
- **Embrace a positive mindset:** Believe in yourself and your ability to achieve your goals.

Remember:

Your Wall Pilates journey is unique. Celebrate your progress, connect with others, and continue exploring the possibilities. Every step you take, every challenge you overcome, contributes to a healthier, happier, and more fulfilling life. Keep moving, keep growing, and keep inspiring yourself and others!

Chapter 14

Beyond Wall Pilates: Additional Resources and Explorations

Congratulations! You've mastered the foundational movements of Wall Pilates and unlocked a world of possibilities for enhancing your fitness and well-being. This chapter delves into **further resources and exploration avenues** to keep you engaged, challenged, and progressing on your journey.

Expanding Your Practice:

- **Explore different Wall Pilates variations:** Discover new exercises targeting specific muscle groups or incorporating equipment like light weights or resistance bands.
- **Join online workouts or classes:** Find virtual instructors offering Wall Pilates

sessions tailored to various fitness levels and goals.

- **Invest in personalized instruction:** Consider working with a certified Wall Pilates instructor for individualized guidance and program design.
- **Explore Pilates variations:** Branch out into mat Pilates or reformer Pilates for a broader range of exercises and challenges.
- **Incorporate other fitness activities:** Cross-train with activities like yoga, swimming, or dancing to add variety and prevent plateaus.

Deepening Your Knowledge:

- **Read books and articles:** Delve into books, articles, and websites dedicated to Wall Pilates and its benefits for various health conditions.
- **Watch instructional videos:** Utilize online video tutorials to refine your technique and learn new exercises.
- **Attend workshops or conferences:** Immerse yourself in the world of Wall

Pilates by attending workshops or conferences led by renowned instructors.

- **Connect with healthcare professionals:** Consult your doctor or physical therapist for personalized advice on integrating Wall Pilates into your overall health plan.

- **Explore the history and philosophy of Pilates:** Gain a deeper appreciation for the practice by understanding its origins and core principles.

Staying Motivated and Inspired:

- **Set new goals:** Challenge yourself with progressive goals, whether increasing workout duration, mastering new exercises, or improving your balance.

- **Track your progress:** Monitor your achievements using journals, fitness trackers, or progress photos to stay motivated and celebrate milestones.

- **Reward yourself:** Acknowledge your efforts with non-food rewards like relaxing spa treatments, new workout gear, or exciting experiences.

- **Share your journey:** Inspire others by sharing your story, progress, and tips on social media or online communities.
- **Find a workout buddy:** Partnering with someone can boost accountability, add fun, and provide support on challenging days.

Remember:

Your fitness journey is an ongoing exploration. Embrace the opportunity to learn, grow, and discover new ways to move your body and optimize your well-being. Wall Pilates is a powerful tool, but it's just the beginning. Keep exploring, keep learning, and keep thriving!

Redefining Your Sixty: A Life of Vitality, Strength, and Joy

Congratulations! You've reached the end of this enriching journey into Wall Pilates and its potential to transform your life after sixty. Throughout this guide, you've explored gentle yet effective exercises, discovered their benefits for your body and mind, and learned valuable tips for building a sustainable practice.

Remember, Wall Pilates is more than just a collection of movements; it's an invitation to **redefine your sixty**. It's an opportunity to reclaim your strength, rediscover your flexibility, and cultivate a deep sense of well-being that empowers you to live a life brimming with vitality, joy, and endless possibilities.

Here are some key takeaways to carry with you:

- **Your body is capable of amazing things, regardless of your age.** Embrace the potential within you and celebrate every step you take towards a healthier, stronger you.

- **Movement is essential for a fulfilling life.** Wall Pilates offers a gentle yet powerful way to stay active, manage pain, and maintain your independence.
- **Small changes can lead to big results.** Start with short, manageable sessions and gradually increase intensity and duration as you build strength and confidence.
- **Listen to your body.** Respect your limits, modify exercises as needed, and prioritize rest and recovery.
- **You are not alone.** Connect with a community of individuals on similar journeys for support, inspiration, and shared experiences.
- **Celebrate your progress.** Every milestone, big or small, is worth acknowledging and appreciating.
- **Most importantly, have fun!** Find joy in the movement, savor the sense of

accomplishment, and embrace the positive impact Wall Pilates has on your life.

Remember, **you are the author of your story**, and every chapter holds the potential for growth, discovery, and joy. Let Wall Pilates be your guide as you write a new chapter filled with strength, vitality, and the vibrant energy that defines a life well-lived at sixty and beyond.

Final Words of Encouragement and Empowerment:

As you conclude this exploration of Wall Pilates and its potential to enrich your life after sixty, remember these closing words of encouragement and empowerment:

You are an inspiration. Stepping onto this path signifies your commitment to **embracing possibility and defying expectations**. Each gentle movement, each conquered challenge, is a testament to your unwavering spirit and resilience.

This is not just about exercise, it's about transformation. As you strengthen your body, you empower your mind, unlocking a newfound sense of confidence and independence. This journey is not confined to the mat, it spills over into every aspect of your life, filling it with vibrant energy and newfound joy.

Remember, age is just a number. Your potential for growth and self-discovery knows no bounds. Embrace the wisdom you've accumulated, the lessons learned, and the strength you've built. Use it to fuel your journey, one graceful movement at a time.

Celebrate the small victories. Don't underestimate the power of each "I did it!" moment. Every conquered exercise, every milestone reached, is a testament to your dedication and deserves to be acknowledged.

Find your tribe. Surround yourself with individuals who share your passion for well-being. Connect with online communities, join local classes, or find a workout buddy. Together, you can motivate, inspire, and celebrate each other's journeys.

Never stop learning. The world of movement is vast and ever-evolving. Embrace new challenges, explore different variations, and continue to learn and grow. Remember, the most exciting chapters of your story are yet to be written.

Most importantly, have fun! Let joy be your guiding light. Find pleasure in the flow of movement, the connection with your body, and the sense of accomplishment that comes with each step forward.

You are strong, capable, and deserving of a life filled with vitality, strength, and joy. Let Wall Pilates be your stepping stone to a future brimming with possibilities. Go forth, embrace the journey, and redefine your sixty with every graceful movement.

Remember, the power is within you.

Glossary of Pilates Terms

Alignment: Proper positioning of the body during exercises to ensure optimal biomechanics and prevent injury.

Breath: Controlled, diaphragmatic breathing used throughout Pilates exercises to support movement and core engagement.

Core: Group of muscles around the torso, including abdominals, obliques, pelvic floor, and lower back, responsible for stability and movement initiation.

Cues: Verbal or visual prompts used to guide movement technique and ensure proper form.

Exhalation (Exhale): Letting out air from the lungs used to engage core muscles and initiate movement.

Footwork: Specific positioning and movement of the feet during exercises for stability and balance.

Imprinting: Pressing the lower back into the mat to engage core muscles and stabilize the spine.

Inhale: Drawing air into the lungs used to lengthen the spine and prepare for movement.

Neutral Pelvis: A balanced position of the pelvis where the front and back are level and there is no tilting.

Neutral Spine: Maintaining a natural curve in the spine without slouching or arching excessively.

Pelvic Tuck: Pulling the lower belly button in and up to engage core muscles and stabilize the pelvis.

Preparation: Initial position before initiating exercise movement.

Reformer: Specialized Pilates equipment with a sliding carriage and springs used for resistance and assisted exercises.

Repetition: Performing an exercise movement a specific number of times.

Set: Performing a number of repetitions consecutively.

Stability: Maintaining proper body alignment and core engagement throughout exercises.

Transition: Smooth and controlled movement between exercise positions.

Triggering: Activating specific muscle groups before initiation of movement.

Variation: Modification of an exercise to increase or decrease difficulty or target specific muscle groups.

Additional Terms:

- **Abduction:** Moving a limb away from the center of the body.
- **Adduction:** Moving a limb towards the center of the body.
- **Extension:** Straightening a joint.

- **Flexion:** Bending a joint.
- **Rotation:** Turning a joint or body part.

Additional Wall Pilates Variations and Modifications:

Here are some additional Wall Pilates variations and modifications to enhance your practice, target specific muscle groups, and cater to different fitness levels:

Warm-up:

- **Arm Circles:** Stand facing the wall with hands shoulder-width apart. Make small circles forward and backward with both arms simultaneously. Modify: Stand further away from the wall for smaller circles or use lighter weights.
- **Leg Swings:** Stand sideways to the wall and hold onto it for support. Swing one leg forward and back, keeping it straight. Repeat with the other leg. Modify: Stand farther from the wall for smaller swings or do seated leg swings.

Core:

- **Side Plank:** Stand sideways to the wall with forearm against it. Lift hips off the ground, forming a straight line from head to heels. Hold for 30 seconds. Modify: Kneel instead of fully planking, or use a pillow under your forearm for more comfort.
- **Bird-Dog:** Start on all fours with hands shoulder-width apart and knees hip-width apart. Extend one arm forward and the opposite leg back, keeping your back flat. Hold for a few breaths. Repeat on the other side. Modify: Keep your knee bent or use a chair for support when extending your arm.

Lower Body:

- **Squats:** Stand with your back against the wall and feet shoulder-width apart. Slide down the wall as if you were going to sit in a chair, then push back up to starting position. Modify: Use a chair for partial squats or hold onto the wall for more stability.

- **Calf Raises:** Stand facing the wall with feet hip-width apart. Rise up onto your toes, then lower back down. Modify: Hold onto the wall for balance or raise only one heel at a time.

Upper Body:

- **Push-ups:** Start in a high plank position with hands shoulder-width apart and feet hip-width apart, leaning against the wall. Lower your chest towards the wall, then push back up to starting position. Modify: Kneel instead of a full plank or do incline push-ups with hands on a higher surface.
- **Shoulder Circles:** Stand facing the wall with arms raised to shoulder height. Make small circles forward and backward with both arms simultaneously. Modify: Use lighter weights or smaller circles for less challenge.

Cool-down:

- **Hamstring Stretch:** Sit on the floor with your back against the wall and legs extended. Reach towards your toes or shins, keeping your back straight. Hold for 30 seconds. Modify: Use a strap or towel to assist reaching your toes.
- **Cat-Cow:** Start on all fours with hands shoulder-width apart and knees hip-width apart. As you inhale, arch your back and look up (cow pose). As you exhale, round your back and tuck your chin towards your chest (cat pose). Flow smoothly between these movements. Modify: Keep your hands flat on the floor or use a pillow for knee support.

Remember:

- **Always listen to your body and modify exercises as needed.**
- **Focus on proper form and controlled movements.**
- **Start with shorter sessions and gradually increase duration and intensity.**

- **Consult a healthcare professional before starting any new exercise program.**

Wall Pilates Workout Log Sheet

Date: [Date of workout]

Workout Focus: [e.g., Core strengthening, Lower body strengthening, Full body routine]

Duration: [Total workout time]

Notes: [Feel free to use this space for any additional notes, such as modifications made, how you felt during the workout, or your goals for the next session]

Additional Tips:

- Use a separate sheet for each workout or dedicate a notebook for your Wall Pilates journey.
- Track your progress by noting down any increases in sets, reps, or modifications used.

- Record how you felt during and after the workout, including any areas of tightness or soreness.
- Use the notes section to personalize your log and set goals for future workouts.
- Consider adding a "Challenge yourself" section where you can write down variations or additional exercises you want to try in the future.

Here are some additional exercises you can add to your log sheet:

- **Standing Wall Pike:** Holds and pulses
- **Wall Leg Swings:** Front & back swings, side leg swings
- **Side Plank with Hip Abduction:** Holds and pulses
- **Single Leg Knee Raise:** Holds and variations
- **Push-ups on Wall:** Modified incline push-ups
- **Tricep Dips with Chair:** Holds and pulses
- **Wall Sit:** Holds and variations

- **Calf Raises on Wall:** Holds and pulses

Remember, consistency is key! Enjoy your Wall Pilates journey and track your progress with this log sheet to see how you're getting stronger and more flexible!

Link for Sample Workout log sheet

https://docs.google.com/spreadsheets/d/1cyUvr m8Na10_t-JoM7DDDFiI4X5eMgRDZ9GQA_T ON7M/edit?usp=drivesdk

Bonus

https://screenpal.com/watch/cZnb2EVdsRi

Video link for tutorials